Low-Carb Diet A Complete Guide To Starting A Low Carb Lifestyle

Introduction

I want to thank you for reading the book, *"Low-Carb Diet A Complete Guide To Starting A Low Carb Lifestyle"*.

This book contains proven steps and strategies on how to lose weight by using a lower carbohydrate strategy.

I want to show you how to implement a low-carb diet that satisfies your taste buds and keeps your stomach feeling full.

Thanks again for reading this book, I hope you enjoy it!

Chapter 1: Brief History of the Low-carb Diet

Carbohydrates are among the macronutrients that the body needs. However, it is also linked to the development of obesity, diabetes and other similar health problems. To reduce the risk of acquiring these diseases, going on a low-carb diet is one of the most recommended steps to follow.

Carbohydrates in the Body

Carbohydrate is a very common macronutrient. It is present in most foods an average person eats. It is present in fruits and starchy vegetables. It is also present in beverages such as milk. Other natural sources of carbohydrates include seeds, nuts, and legumes such as peas, lentils and various kinds of beans.

Baked goods such as cookies, breads and pies are rich in carbohydrates. Pastas, flour tortillas and similar food items are also high in carbohydrates. Processed foods like candies and sweetened drinks and sodas contain additional carbohydrates in the form of simple sugars.

In the body, carbohydrates serve as quick sources of energy. It is also the body's main energy source. Once eaten, carbohydrates are digested much quicker than proteins or fats. Carbohydrates are converted into glucose, which easily enters the bloodstream. Once in the blood, glucose stimulates the liver to release insulin. This hormone helps deliver glucose to the body's tissues where they can be used for various cellular processes. Glucose that was not used by the cells are converted into glycogen and stored in the liver and muscles. Some of the excess glucose are converted into fats.

Carbohydrates that contain fiber are tougher to digest. These have less impact on the body's glucose levels. This type of carbohydrate has other functions in the body beyond being an energy source. It aids in forming bulk in the colon by attracting water and electrolytes. It also binds toxins and other waste products for excretion.

Basics of the Low-carb Diet

A low-carb diet is one that limits the amount of carbohydrates consumed per meal or snack. It heavily cuts back on carbohydrate foods such as fruit, grains and starchy vegetables. It emphasizes on eating more fats and proteins, and a few other non-starchy vegetables. Low-carb diets come in different variations, each with varying types of food restrictions while also limiting carbohydrate intake.

The main purpose of going on a low-carb diet is to achieve weight loss. However, it is also followed as a way to manage or treat certain conditions like diabetes.

By decreasing the intake of carbohydrates, it is also possible to decrease glucose levels. This leads to lower insulin levels. Lower insulin levels mean that the body is stimulated to burn off glucose in the blood and less glucose storage and conversion into fat.

The focus of the diet is on cutting out carbohydrates and eating more proteins such as fish, eggs, poultry and meat. It also includes some vegetables that are non-starchy. The diet excludes most legumes, grains, sweets, breads, pasta, fruits, starchy vegetables and some seeds and nuts. Some variations of the low-carb diet, though, include small amounts of some whole grains, vegetables and fruits.

A typical low-carb diet limits the daily carbohydrate intake to around 60-130 grams. This amount provides around 240-520 calories.

Some variations of this diet restrict carbohydrates during the initial phase and gradually increase it over the next few days. Some variations have very low-carbohydrate intake, which can go as low as 60 grams, or even less.

On the contrary, the recommended carbohydrate intake per day should consist of 45-65% of the total calorie intake per day. For instance, a person who should take 2,000 calories a day should eat 900-1.300 calories from carbohydrates. This would be around 225 to 325 grams.

Foods to eat

As previously mentioned, meals should focus more on eating fats and proteins. Food allowed on low-carb diet includes:

Meats (organic, free range or grass-fed are best)

- Pork

- Lamb

- Beef

- Chicken

Fish (wild-caught ones are best)

- Trout
- Salmon
- Haddock
- Tuna
- Mackerel
- Herring

Vegetables (non-starchy)

- Broccoli
- Carrots
- Spinach
- Leafy greens
- Cauliflower

Fruits

- Apples
- Blueberries
- Oranges

- Pears
- Strawberries

Seeds and Nuts

- Walnuts
- Almonds
- Tree nuts
- Sunflower seeds

High fat dairy

- Butter
- Cheese
- Yogurt
- Heavy cream

Oils and Fats

- Olive oils
- Coconut oil
- Cod fish liver oil
- Butter

- Lard

Eggs (pastured, free range or omega-3 enriched)

Drinks

- Water

- Tea

- Coffee

- Carbonated drinks without any added artificial sweeteners

Depending on your overall body type and health, some carbohydrates maybe included. These are gradually added in the later stages of the diet. Careful observation should be observed when adding these, as some of these may cause a few unwanted effects such as increased carbohydrate cravings.

- Non gluten grains such as oats, rice, and quinoa

- Tubers (starchy vegetables) such as sweet potatoes and potatoes

- Legumes such as black beans, lentils, and pinto beans

In moderation, these foods are allowable while on a low-carb diet:

- Wine – dry wines with no added carbohydrates or sugars

- Dark chocolate- organic and contains at least 70% cocoa

Foods to avoid

Foods to avoid in the low-carb diet include:

- Sugar – in all sources, such as sweeteners and table sugar added to drinks and food (e.g. baked products). Other food products containing sugar that you need to avoid include candies, fruit juices, soft drinks, agave, and ice cream.

- Gluten grains – These are grains that contain gluten such as wheat, rye, barley and spelt. Also, avoid all food products made with these such as pastas and breads.

- Trans fat – These are often found in baked products and processed foods. Trans fat is also available as partially hydrogenated oils or hydrogenated oils. Avoid foods that contain these as well.

- Seed and vegetable oils that are high in omega-6 fatty acid- Omega-6 fatty acids are known to cause a few negative effects on health and should be avoided. Common sources include oils from cottonseed, soybean, safflower, corn, canola, grapeseed and sunflower.

- Artificial sweeteners – These sweeteners include saccharin, aspartame, acesulfame potassium, sucralose and cyclamates.

- Products labeled "Low fat" or "Diet" – These are likely to contain artificial sweeteners and a few other substances that have negative effects on health.

- Processed foods – In general, if a food is manufactured or processed in a factory, then you should avoid eating it.

Chapter 2: Why Eat Less Carbs

There are many reasons why you should go on a low-carb diet. For one thing, carbohydrates (i.e., too much of it) set off a vicious cycle of eating and weight gain. Carbohydrates are digested and converted into glucose. This primarily drives the hormone insulin. High glucose levels in the blood stimulate insulin release. The rapid increase of glucose most often occurs after eating a high carbohydrate meal. Too much glucose leads to the release of large amounts of insulin. This is part of the body's internal homeostatic process to bring everything into balance.

High glucose levels in the blood are dangerous for the body's tissues. To prevent any damage, insulin has to work fast to bring down the glucose levels in the blood rapidly. Insulin functions by allowing more glucose to enter the cells. Once inside the cells, glucose is used to fuel cellular processes. Excess glucose is converted into fats for storage. While this process is efficient, it also produces something undesirable. Too much glucose means a lot of insulin and rapid decline of levels in the blood. This produces a sugar crash. This is the decrease in energy levels, as well as cravings and poor mental functioning, due to the rapid rise and fall of glucose levels.

The body, then, tries to reinstate a normal and steady state of glucose levels by initiating feelings of hunger, so the vicious cycle starts. Eat lots of carbohydrates and after a few hours, you feel hungry again. The hunger cues are actually false hunger. It is just an after effect of the sugar crash. By responding to this kind of hunger, the body gets into a cycle of rapid fat conversion and storing more fats, leading to weight gain.

This condition also makes it hard to lose weight because the body is in a self-preservation mode. Because glucose is quickly removed from the blood, the body sees it as having inadequate available energy. Hence, it conserves its fat stores instead of burning it.

Another negative effect of this cycle is the development of insulin resistance and diabetes. Because of too much and constant high glucose levels (from high carbohydrate meals, sugar crash and frequent eating), the body also produces a lot of insulin. Two things can happen: the cells become resistant to insulin or the pancreas breaks down from too much work.

The cells are not designed to be exposed to any substance- chemical, hormone, etc. They have an intrinsic protective mechanism that shut off the receptor to stop the stimulation from these substances. Hence, prolonged exposure to insulin drives the cells to shut off most of the receptors that normally respond to insulin. This is an attempt to stop glucose entry because the cells already have too much of it. This is called insulin resistance.

As glucose levels continue to increase in the blood and few are entering the cells, the pancreas becomes affected. The pancreas interprets these conditions as producing inadequate amounts of insulin; hence, it stimulates its cells to produce more and more insulin. Just like the other tissues in the body, the cells of the pancreas are not designed to withstand prolonged requirement to produce insulin these cells will eventually give out, leading to low insulin production.

All these conditions lead to the development of diabetes. As the diabetic condition worsens, other tissues and organs in the body start to suffer, too. The vital organs like kidneys, heart and brain begin to suffer damage.

Reasons for Low-carb Diet

Going on a low-carb diet resets the body back to efficient glucose use and insulin production. This is the main benefit that you can achieve from strictly following this diet plan. With this, a whole lot more benefits are obtained as well. Because the body learns to use glucose better, fewer are converted into fats. The body is also trained to burn fat stores to augment its energy needs; hence, this diet promotes weight lose.

High carbohydrate foods are often unhealthy, processed foods. By cutting back on carbohydrates, one learns to adopt better and healthier eating habits. Eating these highly processed foods is one major factor in constant eating, poor energy and poor cognitive functioning. Low-carb diet helps in getting rid of these cravings and tendencies.

What to Expect

During the first few days into the low-carb diet, a few discomforts may be experienced. These are indications that the body is starting to adjust to the change and learns to obtain fuel from proteins and fats. The following are just some of the effects:

- Bad breath (from ketosis, which is often induced by severe carbohydrate restriction to as low as 20 grams per day)

- Headache

- Weakness

- Diarrhea

- Constipation

- Fatigue

In addition, there are risks when going on a low-carb diet. Most carbohydrate-rich foods are also rich in vital nutrients, minerals and vitamins. Cutting these out from the diet may lead to some nutritional deficiencies. It is important to work with a nutritionist and take some supplements to provide the body's nutritional needs.

How low is low-carb?

There is no definite amount or limit as to how low a person can go. It depends on how the body responds. In general, carbohydrate intake is defined as the following:

- Moderate intake: 130 grams to 225 grams

- Low carbohydrate intake: less than 130 grams of carbohydrates per day

- Very low intake: less than 30 grams of carbohydrates per day

Chapter 3: Low-carb Breakfast

Going low-carb for breakfast is a habit that most people find difficult to follow. Loading up on carbohydrates is the way to start mornings for most of the population. The idea is that carbohydrates for breakfast provide the necessary energy to keep going for the entire morning. According to the low-carb diet, carbohydrates in the morning actually contribute to energy crash by mid-morning.

Notice that by 10 in the morning, your energy level and focus tend to drop. People need to boost themselves with a cup of coffee or a high carbohydrate snack. This is because of the sugar crash that follows a high-carbohydrate breakfast meal. By reducing carbohydrates and eating more fats and proteins to start the day, energy levels are more stable, keeping the body going longer without the need for an energy boost.

Eggs

These are among the most versatile breakfast staples. Omit the toast and fry up some eggs. Make sunny side eggs, eggs Benedict, eggs Florentine, devilled, eggs or scrambled eggs. Go fancier with omelets and frittatas, or just boil some water and have soft-boiled or hard-boiled eggs for breakfast. Are you constantly in a hurry? Place eggs in a bowl of water and pop in the microwave. You can also make the eggs ahead and store them in your refrigerator.

Frittatas

To make breakfast eggs even more convenient, make vegetable frittatas ahead. Cut into serving portions and place in the freezer or refrigerator. Take them out at breakfast and heat in the microwave or pan. Frittatas are basically a cross between a quiche and an omelet, but without the quiche's crust. You can add any kind of vegetable. This is also a good way to use any leftover vegetables. The best thing is that these are quick and easy to make.

Scrambled eggs

Quick and easy. Crack some eggs in a bowl and whisk away. To make things less monotonous, add a few splashes of milk and/or some cheese.

Omelets

These are perfect in using leftovers. Make things more interesting by adding a few meat pieces with some cutup vegetable. Add some herbs, too to amp the health benefits.

Cereals

These can be difficult to work with into the low-carb diet. Most cereals naturally contain large amounts of carbohydrates. There are ways to still get cereals for breakfast, but still stay low-carb.

- Cold cereals have low-carb varieties. Look for these specially labeled products such as Special K.

- Purchase cold cereals that are high in fiber.

- Some cereals are available in special low-carb varieties, such as Flax-O-Meal.

Breads

Breads are breakfast staples that are high in carbohydrates because these are traditionally made from wheat flour. However, there are alternatives that can fit into the low-carb diet, such as muffins and breads made from almond meal, flax meal and other similar low-carb ingredients.

Puddings

Puddings are very filling, yet low-carb breakfast options. These are also quick and easy to make for those busy mornings. One recipe to try is this:

Blueberry and Almond Pudding

Ingredients

- 1/3 cup of almond meal

- ¼ cup of blueberries (fresh or frozen)

- 1 large egg

- 2 tablespoons of water

- Sweeteners (e.g., sugar-free maple syrup, etc.)

- Add-ons (see list at the end of the recipe)

How to prepare

- Combine egg, water and almond meal in a small saucepan. Cook over medium high heat for 2 to 3 minutes. Add the blueberries in the middle of the mixture and cook on low heat. Remove from heat once pudding is set and firm. Stir to mix berries well before serving.

<u>Additions (optional)</u>

- Unsweetened coconut

- Cream cheese, cut into small cubes

- Nut butters such as peanut butter

- Chopped nuts

- Sugar-free preserves or jams

Yogurt, ricotta and cottage cheese

These spoonable dairy products can be quick, filling, healthy, low-carb breakfast items. Add nuts, flax seed or some fresh or frozen low-carb fruits.

Shakes and smoothies

Shakes and smoothies are quick, nutrient-packed breakfast on the go. Add protein powders, soymilk (unsweetened), water or kefir to yogurt or cheese (ricotta, cream cheese) and blend in a food processor or blender.

Tofu

Soft tofu is a good rich source of protein. It can be added to smoothies or eat it as it is with a spoonful of berries or cheeses. You can cut up hard tofu into smaller pieces and add them to omelets, frittatas or tofu scrambles.

Chapter 4: Low-carb Lunch

Lunch is often synonymous to sandwiches. Most people eat lunch on the go, while running errands or doing some work at their desks or in front of a computer terminal. Low-carb lunch can still fit right into busy schedules and still have enough energy to last through the rest of a hectic day.

Salads

If eggs are low-carb breakfast best buddies, salads are to lunch. Go beyond the traditional chef's salad of hard-boiled eggs, cheese, cold cuts over greens. The kinds of salads that you can include in your low-carb lunch meal plan are only limited to your imagination.

Iceberg lettuce is traditionally part of any salad. Switch it with different types of greens such as spinach and other lettuce varieties like red sails and Romaine and because of the growing popularity of salads of late, there are already premixed bagged salad greens in groceries and supermarkets. Just open and add a drizzle of low-carb dressing.

A few examples of salads and add-ons that fit right into a low-carb diet include:

- Greek salad with added proteins like shrimps, chicken or hard-boiled eggs

- Low-carb taco salad

- Thai-style chicken salad

- Salad with chicken (pan fried without breading), leafy greens, red peppers, walnuts and snow pea pods.

- Cole slaw with diced apples and chicken, topped with roasted pecans

- Tuna salad (steamed tuna, flaked, with dressing of choice), mixed with slices of avocado and tomatoes, and some leafy greens

- Grilled salmon on a bed of leafy salad greens, mushrooms, sprouts and blanched green beans

- Steamed chicken breast, cubed, and mixed with cucumber slices and greens, topped with crumbled blue cheese and toasted pecans

- Grilled steak with a siding of greens, mushrooms, green peppers and red onions (sliced thinly)

- Cob salad

Low-carbohydrate Taco Salad

Ingredients

- 1 pound of ground beef

- 1 tablespoon of chili powder (adjusted according to taste)

- 8 pieces of green onions, chopped, separate piles for green and white parts

- Pepper and salt, according to preference

- 1 medium-sized tomato, diced

- 1 head of romaine lettuce, sliced

- 1 medium avocado, diced

- Ripe olives, optional, sliced or chopped

- ½ cup of salsa

- ½ cup of sour cream

- 1 ½ cups of grated cheese- may be Monterey Jack, cheddar or combination of different cheeses

How to prepare

- Place skillet over high heat and add beef. Cook until no longer pink. Remove any excess liquids. Add chili powder and the sliced white parts of the onions. Season according to preference with pepper and salt. Remove from heat and set aside. Add to salad warm or cold, according to preference.

- In a separate bowl, combine green part of the onions, olives (I using), avocado, tomato and lettuce. Toss. Add the cheeses and meat if desired, or keep the salad, cheese and meat in separate layers.

- Top the salad with salsa and some sour cream.

Dressings

Dressings are easy to make. There are vinaigrettes and creamy, low-carb dressings. Bottled ones are used with caution, though. Some of these have hidden carbohydrates. Diet or light dressings are also not recommended because most have added sugars to compensate for flavor loss due to reduced fat contents.

Dressings should be high in monounsaturated fats, for example, olive oil. These help in making salads more filling and satisfying. These fats are also high in health benefits such as protective effects on the heart and decreased cholesterol levels in the blood.

Oil-based dressings are best to use and easy to make. It takes less than 1 minute to make, in fact. Just mix a few tablespoons of olive oil, add a few drops of apple cider vinegar, freshly squeezed lemon juice, and some herbs. Whisk in a bowl and add salad vegetables on top. Toss to coat everything well.

Creamy dressings are safest when homemade. Ingredients are sure to be low-carb with no added sugars. Mix yogurt with lemon juice and herbs, or mix mayonnaise with spices and herbs, thinned down with lemon juice or water.

Greek Salad Dressing with Lemon and Garlic

Ingredients

- ¾ cup of extra virgin olive oil

- ¼ cup of freshly squeezed lemon juice

- 2 teaspoons Greek oregano or Greek seasoning

- ½ teaspoon of salt

- 1 teaspoon of Dijon mustard

- Ground pepper, optional and according to taste

- 2 cloves of garlic, finely minced grated or pressed

How to prepare

- Mix everything in a bowl or glass jar.

- If using a bowl, whisk everything while adding the olive oil in a thin and steady stream.

- If using a jar, add olive oil last, cover tightly and shake well.

- Taste and adjust according to preference. Add more olive oil to reduce acidity. Add more lemon juice if more acidity is preferred.

Wraps and roll ups

Low-carb roll up lunches come in three main varieties:

Lettuce

Lettuce is used to wrap mushy foods such as egg, chicken, salmon or tuna salad. Choose larger leaves for better and fuller cover of the fillings. Add vegetables to the fillings, such as strips of cucumber, carrots or bell pepper.

Meat

Meat roll ups are simple, filling, low-carb lunch options. Roll vegetables slices and cheese on a slice of bacon, ham, chicken breast, roast beef, etc. The options are endless. You may also use salads as fillings. For example, spoon some coleslaw over ham slices and carefully roll.

Low-carb Tortillas

Most tortillas are flour-based and high in carbohydrates. It is important to choose low-carb tortillas. Wrap anything with these, such as salads, meats and cheeses.

Soups

These are versatile meal options. Add leftover meats and vegetables for a whole new meal item. Most soups are already low in carb. Just make sure to limit adding starchy vegetables. Also, omit using flour and similar carbohydrate-rich thickeners.

Canned soups are often high in carbohydrates, from thickeners, stabilizers, additives, flavorings and preservatives. Read labels well to be certain that canned soups are indeed low-carb before purchasing or using.

Too, make it easier and more convenient to serve soups by setting aside some time to make a huge pot. Cool and ladle into serving portions in separate containers. Freeze.

Leftovers

It is not required to cook or prepare different foods for every meal. Recycle leftovers. In fact, you can use leftovers from your prepared dinner to cut down cooking and preparation time for succeeding meals. For example, instead of making dinner enough for yourself (and some dinner company), add a serving or two and set it aside for tomorrow's breakfast or lunch.

Chapter 5: Low-carb Dinner

Most main dishes are naturally low in carbohydrates, as these are mainly meat, poultry or seafood dishes. A few adjustments are all it takes to make dinners even lower in carbohydrate contents. To keep planning simpler, think of favorite main dishes. Start with a menu that includes proteins cooked in plain and simple ways such as pan-grilled salmon, steamed chicken, grilled steak, broiled fish, and pan-fried chicken.

For usual fares of rice or pasta, substitute these with more servings of vegetables. To make it look more enticing, use several colored-vegetables. Mix leafy greens with bright colors of bell peppers (yellow and red), carrots, beets and the like. Also, add some spices to make it more interesting to the palate, such as a dash of cayenne or turmeric. Add more healthy forms of fats like a drizzle of olive oil to help increase satiety from meals.

Try new cuisines. Turn a carb-restrictive diet into a palate adventure. Many foreign cuisines are in fact, naturally low in carbohydrates. Try Asian cuisines such as Thai and Indian. Leave out the rice and noodles and go for more of the stir-frys and meat dishes. Thai cuisine is rich in delicious and varied vegetable dishes. Indian cuisine is high in meats and spices that promise to be an explosion of flavors. Traditional Greek cooking is more on vegetables, too and with lots of healthy fats from olive oils and fish dishes. Traditional French cooking contains moderate amounts of carbohydrates.

Thai Curry Chicken in Coconut Milk

Ingredients

- 1 pound of chicken thighs or breast, sliced into bite size

- 1 can of coconut milk

- 1 red bell pepper, diced

- ½ of a medium-sized onion, diced

- 12 ounces of frozen or fresh green beans

- Thai spices, adjusted according to taste

How to prepare

- Heat olive or coconut oil in a pan over medium high heat.

- Add the onions and pepper. Cook until onions are soft and translucent.

- Add Thai spices. Season according to preference with pepper and salt. Keep stirring and cooking until the spices start to smell fragrant.

- Add sliced chicken. Stir until the chicken is almost cooked through.

- Pour the coconut milk and bring the entire mixture to a boil. Lower the heat to a simmer and continue cooking for 3-5 minutes more.

Chapter 6: Low-carb Snacks and Desserts

Snacks and desserts are often the most difficult to deal with on a low-carb diet. Most desserts are made with flour, which is high in carbohydrates not to mention, most desserts are also full of sugar. Snacks are the same. On a low-carb diet, these are often the first ones to go.

Most people are unaware that snack and desserts go beyond the usual high carbohydrate options. There are vegetables (non-starchy) and dips that are filling snacks, packed with nutrients but low on carbohydrates. There are flourless and sugar-free versions of favorite desserts, too.

Sugar-free Jell-O

These are perfect as dessert or snack. These come in ready to eat snack cups. These can also be used in whipping up a good, delicious dessert low in carbohydrates. Add some whipped cream to make it more interesting.

Peanuts

These are perfect, convenient snacks. Peanuts are protein-rich, low in carbohydrate, rich in healthy fats. It is also rich in fiber, which further reduces the net carbs you get. There is just about 3.6 net carbs for 28 pieces of peanuts.

Sugar-free Popsicles

Sugar-free popsicles can help get those cravings at bay. Bonus point in eating these cold treats is that the mouth becomes really cold. This will prevent you from thinking of food or wanting to eat for quite a while when you are done with one.

Almonds

Like peanuts, almonds are perfect snack treats. Munch on these when you are craving, or in need of an energy boost. Eating 24 whole pieces of almonds can provide only 2.3 net carbs.

Dill pickles

About three big slices of dill pickles provide only 1 carbohydrate. Dill pickles do not contain any sugar, compared to sweet pickles.

Grapes

Per 10 pieces of grapes, you only get about 8.5 net carbohydrates. A handful is good, but make sure that you do not go overboard. Grapes still contain sugar in them and it is easy to eat too much.

Lemon

Raw lemons can be good for snacks. It is especially good on days when you are craving for something sweet. Sucking on lemon slices can get those sweet thoughts off or you can just make lemon water to sip throughout the day. It helps keep you hydrated and boost the energy. Squeeze about half a lemon into a small bottle of water.

Strawberries

For 8 pieces of strawberries, you get about six net carbohydrates. Eat a few pieces as dessert to satisfy the sweet tooth, but still within the carbohydrate limitations.

Eggs

These may be more part of a meal than a snack. However, eggs can be great as energy boosters and drive away cravings.

Cheese

Tasty, filling, and low on carbohydrates. Keep a few slices with you to munch on when you need a quick snack or when you start craving.

Other snack ideas:

- Celery sticks with peanut butter dip

- Celery sticks with tuna salad dip

- Deviled or hard-boiled eggs

- Berries and cheese (mix ¼ cup of fresh or frozen berries and 1/3 cup of cottage cheese)

- Sunflower, pumpkin or squash seeds

- Trail mix (low-carb variety)

- Turkey or beef jerky, low-sugar variety

- String cheese and other cheese sticks

- Toasted pepperoni slices

- Apple slices with some cheese

- Yogurt (sugar-free) with flax seed and berries

- Roll-ups, such as lettuce with egg salad or luncheon meat

- Cucumber slices, with cream cheese and smoked salmon

- Vegetables (such as lettuce, carrot sticks, celery, cucumber) with bean dip or spinach dip

- Crispy pork rinds

- Mushrooms stuffed with cheese spread or other low-carb dips

- Fruits and nuts with ricotta cheese

- Peanut butter protein bars or balls

- Parmesan crisps

Low Carb Cheesecake

<u>Ingredients</u>

- 3 packages of cream cheese, at room temperature

- 4 large eggs, at room temperature

- 1 ½ teaspoon of lemon juice, freshly squeezed

- 1 ½ teaspoon vanilla

- ¼ cup of sour cream

- 1 1/3 cups of Stevia

For the crust

- 2 tablespoon of butter, melted

- 1 cup of almond meal

- 2 tablespoon of Stevia

How to prepare

- Prepare the oven by heating it at 375 degrees Fahrenheit.

- Mix the ingredients for the crust. Press it firmly into a spring form pan. Bake in the oven for about 8-10 minutes, until the crust starts to turn brown and fragrant. Remove from the oven and set aside to cool.

- Increase the oven heat to 400 degrees Fahrenheit.

- In a mixing bowl, place cream cheese. Beat with a hand mixer until it becomes fluffy. Add all the other ingredients while beating. Scrape the sides of the bowl towards the center to incorporate everything well. Once well combined, scrape from the sides of the bowl and toward the center one last time. Beat for another minute.

- Pour the cheesecake mixture over the prepared crust.

- Bake in the oven in a water bath. For the water bath, get some aluminum foil and wrap it all over the sides and bottom of pan. Place it in a deep baking pan and pour some boiling water around the side of the springform pan. Bake the cheesecake at 350 degrees Fahrenheit, for 60-90 minutes. Remove the cheesecake from the oven once the cake is firm when touched, but still slightly soft in the center.

- Chill and top with some fruits.

Raspberry Jelly Squares

Ingredients

- 1 package (about 3 ounces) of gelatin dessert, sugar-free and raspberry flavored

- 1 ½ cups of boiling water

- 2 tablespoons of butter

- 1 cup of pecans

- ¼ cup of Stevia

- A pinch of salt

- 6 ounces of cream cheese, cut into small pieces

- 1 ½ cups of raspberries, fresh or frozen (unsweetened)

- ¼ teaspoon of orange extract

How to prepare

- Prepare the oven by heating to 350 degrees Fahrenheit.

- Open the gelatin pack and pour into a bowl with the boiling water. Dissolve and set aside.

- Place the pecans in a food processor and process until it resembles a coarse meal.

- Add salt, Stevia and butter into the food processor, and continue processing until the mixture has a smooth consistency.

- Remove the pecan mixture. Press into a pan, making it as a base for the dessert. Bake in the preheated oven until the pecan crust turns light brown, for about 8 to 11 minutes. Remove from the oven and set aside.

- Check the gelatin, if it is comfortably warm enough to stick a finger into it. Place it in a blender and add cream cheese and orange extract. Blend until smooth and even in consistency. Remove and add a cup of berries. Mix and pour over the crust.

- Place in the refrigerator and chill for 10 to 20 minutes, until the raspberry gelatin mixture has thickened but not yet set. Add ½ cup of raspberries on top of the mixture and return to the refrigerator.

- Cool until the mixture has completely set. Cut into squares and serve or store in airtight containers.

Chapter 7: Low-carb Diet Tips and Suggestions

In the low-carb diet, one of the biggest difficulties to sustaining this diet is boredom. In most people, boredom is a result of inadequate knowledge and poor understanding of the diet. Most people become overwhelmed by the restriction on practically most of the foods they used to enjoy. Take note that in the recommended nutrition intake, carbohydrates are only about 45 to 50% of the calories. However, an average person consumes a lot more than this. Granted, an average person's favorite foods are rich in carbohydrates.

However, there are a whole lot more to food than just those carbohydrates. There are filling, satisfying, comforting foods that are in carbohydrates. Flavorful foods are not only those high in carbohydrates. Desserts, sweet indulgences and snacks are also not just limited to carbohydrates.

To make low-carb diet less boring and more exciting, try these tips and tricks:

Give more attention to the kinds of foods that you are allowed to eat, instead of dwelling on the restrictions.

Dwelling on things that are no longer part of the diet is a huge setback to achieving success in low-carb diet, or any other diet for that matter. Carbohydrates are just a part of an entire world of food. There is a long list of meats, different kinds of fishes and seafood, eggs, vegetables (some), fruits (some), dairy products (yogurt, various kinds of cheeses), seeds, nuts (and products made from them such as nut butters and milks), oils and a lot other healthy sources of fats.

Find how much carbohydrates fit your needs and lifestyle

The body needs carbohydrates. Problems only arise if there is too much intake and from unhealthy sources. Going low-carb does not have to be too restricted. It all depends on how the body responds. One person may eat as low as 30 grams per day and still be fine. Another person can go as much as 125 grams per day and still lose weight and achieve other health benefits. The key is to find what works best for you.

In finding the right carbohydrate count, things to consider would be the highest carbohydrate intake and still achieve:

1. Weight loss or maintain current weight

2. Absence of cravings for high-carb food

Cravings are very important markers that determine if the carbohydrate intake should be increased or reduced. If a person gets cravings when increasing carbohydrate intake by a few grams, it means the body cannot tolerate that particular amount. Lower it until the body is no longer raving. This is the hallmark that one has already achieved the optimum healthy carbohydrate intake.

Other signs that the optimum carbohydrate level is already achieved include:

- Increased mental alertness

- Improved energy levels

- Better blood glucose level (for pre-diabetics and diabetics)

Be more adventurous with food by trying out new cuisines.

There is an entire world of different cuisines. In each cuisine, there are lots of recipes that are naturally low in carbohydrates.

Find "de-carbed" version of favorite foods

With the growing awareness of carbohydrates and their effects, there are now de-carbed versions of most foods. There are now de-carbed pizza and cakes. Omitting sugar and choosing healthier sugar substitutes like Stevia works in reducing carbohydrates, too.

Learn how to cook

Start with simple and easy to make meals. Salads are pretty easy to make. Do not go for gourmet if you are still starting to learn how to cook to avoid getting overwhelmed. However, before cooking your own meals, it is more important to have a good understanding of the diet. Getting familiar with foods to eat and not to eat would take some time and effort. Learning to cook low-carb would also take quite some time to get used to.

Re-assess yourself

Sometimes, boredom is not really boredom. It is more of feeling deprived because you have not had your favorite foods for quite some time, or there might be a few other issues about the diet. Take a step back and re-assess yourself. Find out what it is that hinders you from embracing the low-carb lifestyle fully. Address it head-on.

If the concern is missing your old-time favorites, include eating a small portion of it in your meal plan. When planning your weekly menu, set aside a certain time of the week to eat your favorite food. For example, include half a slice of chocolate cake for dessert on Wednesday nights, or have half a slice of pizza on Friday evenings. Make adjustments to the rest of the day's carbohydrate intake on days you plan to eat your favorite high carb food. This way, you do not get deprived and feel depressed about the diet limitations.

Common Mistakes to Avoid on the Low-Card Diet

Starting improperly

Starting on the wrong foot is a recipe for failure. Good thing is you do not have to get a college degree to understand carbohydrates. Most people think that going low carb means eating meats and fats all day. There is more to this diet than just that. This is why it is important to know and understand the food list.

Giving up too soon

Going low carb after years of enjoying high carbohydrate foods like cakes, pastas and breads is difficult. The body has learned to depend on carbohydrates for fuel and it may take some time before it learns to use fuel provided by proteins and fats. Most people give up too soon, especially when difficulties arise or when weight loss is not proceeding as desired.

Understand that there is no standard on how low you should go on this diet. It all depends on your body's needs and response to the diet. There will be missteps. You will have to deal with cravings. You will fall off the wagon. You will eat more carbohydrates at times than what you intend to. These are all part of the process in finding the right carbohydrate amount for you. The point is not in avoiding these mistakes. These are actually crucial in determining how much you can tolerate to determine how much you should take. These are not indications that you should just give up. These are indications that you must keep going to get the best results.

Not eating enough vegetables

Vegetables are very important in the success of this kind of diet. Too little vegetables on a protein-rich and high-fat diet could lead to constipation, bloating, gas and a few other discomforts. You can avoid these by adding more fiber through more vegetables.

Not eating enough fat

Fats are important on this diet because these help in making a meal satisfying and more filling. The problem is there is still a huge misconception about fats in the diet. Not all fats are bad. There are healthy fats that should be added to the diet, such as omega-3 fats from cold-water fishes and monounsaturated fats from olive oil.

Adding fats is also important in losing weight on the low-carb diet. It helps provide energy. Too little fats can actually lead to weight gain even while on a restricted diet and regular exercise. The body feels as if it is deprived of energy (starvation), which leads to more fat conversion of protein and carbohydrates. By adding more fats to the diet, the body is assured that it will have a steady supply of fuel, and it is all right to keep burning its fat stores.

Not eating enough fiber

As has been previously mentioned, fiber helps in preventing some of the discomforts of eating more proteins and fats, and eating small amounts of carbohydrates. These can be obtained in leafy greens, as well as some non-starchy vegetables.

Eating too much

The good thing about low-carb diet is that there is no need to count calories. This is both a good thing and a bad one. Some people think that by limiting carbohydrate intake, they can already eat unlimited amounts of proteins and fats and still achieve their weight loss goals. Eating more than what the body needs- whether carbohydrates, fats or proteins- will still lead to weight gain. The best guide is to eat when hungry and stop when comfortably full.

Not enough planning

Diets require a plan. Meal plans are important because they serve as a guide on what you should eat at certain times of the day. This way, you avoid inadvertently going for a high-carbohydrate take-out meal or snack. It reduces the routine, mindless drive-throughs and trips to the vending machine. Sitting down and making a meal plan is also a time to stop, re-assess eating habits and make better decisions when it comes to food.

It is difficult to make healthy decisions when you are tired or stressed, or even when you are happy and excited about something. Emotions often get in the way and soon, you catch yourself munching on cookies or eating a tub of ice cream. With a meal plan, you know exactly what you should be eating, regardless of what emotional state you are in. It is also a good reminder to stick to the diet whenever you are starting to slide back to old habits.

Experiencing a rut

Everyone gets into a rut at some point, even the most determined and most disciplined of dieters. This is most often due to poor meal planning, eating the same things every single day. Salads every day for an entire week is a good way to get into a rut. Spice things up and introduce new foods from time to time. Switch meal schedules, such as eating salads meats at lunch and salads for dinner. Instead of fresh green salad, make one with grilled vegetables. Try new dishes from different cuisines. Sometimes, as simple as adding a few new herbs or spices in your usual fare can help get rid of boredom.

Packaged low-carb foods

There is a new aisle of special low-carb foods nowadays- from cereals to ice creams and other treats. It is very tempting to take the easier way of just buying these packaged stuff instead of cooking and preparing your own meals at home.

However, be very wary when buying these packaged low-carb food items. These often contain chemical substitutes that do much worse things in the body than regular sugar and carbohydrates do. For example, the chemical maltitol is a common sugar substitute known to have negative effects in the body.

Carb creep

Most people fall off the diet because of carb creep. This is the slow, unnoticed increase in carbohydrate intake. Adding a little carbohydrate may not give any noticeable effects until one day, you wake up with the worst carb craving. Carb creep is oftentimes subtle, until after you notice that you are no longer feeling as great as you were when you started on the diet and you start gaining weight. Watch out for carb creep and constantly monitor how your body responds to keep within your limits.

Conclusion

Thank you again for reading this book!

I hope you are on your way to a healthier you.